IF FOUND, PLEASE RETURN THIS PLANNER TO:

_____

_____

_____

_____

_____

2020 AT A GLANCE

JANUARY
S	M	T	W	T	F	S
			1	2	3	4
5	6	7	8	9	10	11
12	13	14	15	16	17	18
19	20	21	22	23	24	25
26	27	28	29	30	31	

FEBRUARY
S	M	T	W	T	F	S
						1
2	3	4	5	6	7	8
9	10	11	12	13	14	15
16	17	18	19	20	21	22
23	24	25	26	27	28	29

MARCH
S	M	T	W	T	F	S
1	2	3	4	5	6	7
8	9	10	11	12	13	14
15	16	17	18	19	20	21
22	23	24	25	26	27	28
29	30	31				

APRIL
S	M	T	W	T	F	S
			1	2	3	4
5	6	7	8	9	10	11
12	13	14	15	16	17	18
19	20	21	22	23	24	25
26	27	28	29	30		

MAY
S	M	T	W	T	F	S
					1	2
3	4	5	6	7	8	9
10	11	12	13	14	15	16
17	18	19	20	21	22	23
24	25	26	27	28	29	30
31						

JUNE
S	M	T	W	T	F	S
	1	2	3	4	5	6
7	8	9	10	11	12	13
14	15	16	17	18	19	20
21	22	23	24	25	26	27
28	29	30				

JULY
S	M	T	W	T	F	S
			1	2	3	4
5	6	7	8	9	10	11
12	13	14	15	16	17	18
19	20	21	22	23	24	25
26	27	28	29	30	31	

AUGUST
S	M	T	W	T	F	S
						1
2	3	4	5	6	7	8
9	10	11	12	13	14	15
16	17	18	19	20	21	22
23	24	25	26	27	28	29
30	31					

SEPTEMBER
S	M	T	W	T	F	S
		1	2	3	4	5
6	7	8	9	10	11	12
13	14	15	16	17	18	19
20	21	22	23	24	25	26
27	28	29	30			

OCTOBER
S	M	T	W	T	F	S
				1	2	3
4	5	6	7	8	9	10
11	12	13	14	15	16	17
18	19	20	21	22	23	24
25	26	27	28	29	30	31

NOVEMBER
S	M	T	W	T	F	S
1	2	3	4	5	6	7
8	9	10	11	12	13	14
15	16	17	18	19	20	21
22	23	24	25	26	27	28
29	30					

DECEMBER
S	M	T	W	T	F	S
		1	2	3	4	5
6	7	8	9	10	11	12
13	14	15	16	17	18	19
20	21	22	23	24	25	26
27	28	29	30	31		

2021 AT A GLANCE

JANUARY

S	M	T	W	T	F	S
					1	2
3	4	5	6	7	8	9
10	11	12	13	14	15	16
17	18	19	20	21	22	23
24	25	26	27	28	29	30
31						

FEBRUARY

S	M	T	W	T	F	S
	1	2	3	4	5	6
7	8	9	10	11	12	13
14	15	16	17	18	19	20
21	22	23	24	25	26	27
28	29					

MARCH

S	M	T	W	T	F	S
	1	2	3	4	5	6
7	8	9	10	11	12	13
14	15	16	17	18	19	20
21	22	23	24	25	26	27
28	29	30	31			

APRIL

S	M	T	W	T	F	S
				1	2	3
4	5	6	7	8	9	10
11	12	13	14	15	16	17
18	19	20	21	22	23	24
25	26	27	28	29	30	

MAY

S	M	T	W	T	F	S
						1
2	3	4	5	6	7	8
9	10	11	12	13	14	15
16	17	18	19	20	21	22
23	24	25	26	27	28	29
30	31					

JUNE

S	M	T	W	T	F	S
		1	2	3	4	5
6	7	8	9	10	11	12
13	14	15	16	17	18	19
20	21	22	23	24	25	26
27	28	29	30			

JULY

S	M	T	W	T	F	S
				1	2	3
4	5	6	7	8	9	10
11	12	13	14	15	16	17
18	19	20	21	22	23	24
25	26	27	28	29	30	31

AUGUST

S	M	T	W	T	F	S
1	2	3	4	5	6	7
8	9	10	11	12	13	14
15	16	17	18	19	20	21
22	23	24	25	26	27	28
29	30	31				

SEPTEMBER

S	M	T	W	T	F	S
			1	2	3	4
5	6	7	8	9	10	11
12	13	14	15	16	17	18
19	20	21	22	23	24	25
26	27	28	29	30		

OCTOBER

S	M	T	W	T	F	S
					1	2
3	4	5	6	7	8	9
10	11	12	13	14	15	16
17	18	19	20	21	22	23
24	25	26	27	28	29	30
31						

NOVEMBER

S	M	T	W	T	F	S
	1	2	3	4	5	6
7	8	9	10	11	12	13
14	15	16	17	18	19	20
21	22	23	24	25	26	27
28	29	30				

DECEMBER

S	M	T	W	T	F	S
			1	2	3	4
5	6	7	8	9	10	11
12	13	14	15	16	17	18
19	20	21	22	23	24	25
26	27	28	29	30	31	

CONTACTS

NAME	ADDRESS/ NUMBERS

CONTACTS

NAME	ADDRESS/ NUMBERS

CONTACTS

NAME	ADDRESS/ NUMBERS

CONTACTS

NAME	ADDRESS/ NUMBERS

JANUARY

Sunday	Monday	Tuesday	Wednesday
			1
5	6	7	8
12	13	14	15
19	20	21	22
26	27	28	29

2020

Thursday	Friday	Saturday	Notes
2	**3**	**4**	
9	**10**	**11**	
16	**17**	**18**	
23	**24**	**25**	
30	**31**		**FEBRUARY**

FEBRUARY

S	M	T	W	T	F	S
						1
2	3	4	5	6	7	8
9	10	11	12	13	14	15
16	17	18	19	20	21	22
23	24	25	26	27	28	29

JANUARY 2020

MONDAY
30

TUESDAY
31

WEDNESDAY
1

THURSDAY
2

FRIDAY

3

SATURDAY

4

SUNDAY

5

WEEKLY GOALS

JANUARY 2020

MONDAY

6

TUESDAY

7

WEDNESDAY

8

THURSDAY

9

JANUARY 2020

FRIDAY
10

SATURDAY
11

SUNDAY
12

WEEKLY GOALS

JANUARY 2020

MONDAY

13

TUESDAY

14

WEDNESDAY

15

THURSDAY

16

JANUARY 2020

FRIDAY
17

SATURDAY
18

SUNDAY
19

WEEKLY GOALS

JANUARY 2020

MONDAY
20

TUESDAY
21

WEDNESDAY
22

THURSDAY
23

FRIDAY
24

SATURDAY
25

SUNDAY
26

WEEKLY GOALS

JANUARY 2020

MONDAY
27

TUESDAY
28

WEDNESDAY
29

THURSDAY
30

FEBRUARY 2020

FRIDAY

31

SATURDAY

1

SUNDAY

2

WEEKLY GOALS

FEBRUARY

Sunday	Monday	Tuesday	Wednesday
2	3	4	5
9	10	11	12
16	17	18	19
23	24	25	26

2020

Thursday	Friday	Saturday	Notes
		1	
6	**7**	**8**	
13	**14**	**15**	
20	**21**	**22**	**JANUARY**
27	**28**	**29**	**MARCH**

JANUARY

S	M	T	W	T	F	S
			1	2	3	4
5	6	7	8	9	10	11
12	13	14	15	16	17	18
19	20	21	22	23	24	25
26	27	28	29	30	31	

MARCH

S	M	T	W	T	F	S
1	2	3	4	5	6	7
8	9	10	11	12	13	14
15	16	17	18	19	20	21
22	23	24	25	26	27	28
29	30	31				

FEBRUARY 2020

MONDAY

3

TUESDAY

4

WEDNESDAY

5

THURSDAY

6

FRIDAY
7

SATURDAY
8

SUNDAY
9

WEEKLY GOALS

FEBRUARY 2020

MONDAY

10

TUESDAY

11

WEDNESDAY

12

THURSDAY

13

FEBRUARY 2020

FRIDAY
14

SATURDAY
15

SUNDAY
16

WEEKLY GOALS

FEBRUARY 2020

MONDAY
17

TUESDAY
18

WEDNESDAY
19

THURSDAY
20

FRIDAY
21

SATURDAY
22

SUNDAY
23

WEEKLY GOALS

FEBRUARY 2020

MONDAY

24

TUESDAY

25

WEDNESDAY

26

THURSDAY

27

FRIDAY

28

SATURDAY

29

SUNDAY

1

WEEKLY GOALS

MARCH

Sunday	Monday	Tuesday	Wednesday
1	2	3	4
8	9	10	11
15	16	17	18
22	23	24	25
29	30	31	

Thursday	Friday	Saturday	Notes
5	**7**	**7**	
12	**13**	**14**	
19	**20**	**21**	
26	**27**	**28**	

FEBRUARY

S	M	T	W	T	F	S
						1
2	3	4	5	6	7	8
9	10	11	12	13	14	15
16	17	18	19	20	21	22
23	24	25	26	27	28	29

APRIL

S	M	T	W	T	F	S
			1	2	3	4
5	6	7	8	9	10	11
12	13	14	15	16	17	18
19	20	21	22	23	24	25
26	27	28	29	30		

MARCH 2020

MONDAY

2

TUESDAY

3

WEDNESDAY

4

THURSDAY

5

FRIDAY

6

SATURDAY

7

SUNDAY

8

WEEKLY GOALS

MARCH 2020

MONDAY
9

TUESDAY
10

WEDNESDAY
11

THURSDAY
12

FRIDAY
13

SATURDAY
14

SUNDAY
15

WEEKLY GOALS

MARCH 2020

MONDAY
16

TUESDAY
17

WEDNESDAY
18

THURSDAY
19

FRIDAY

20

SATURDAY

21

SUNDAY

22

WEEKLY GOALS

MARCH 2020

MONDAY
23

TUESDAY
24

WEDNESDAY
25

THURSDAY
26

FRIDAY
27

SATURDAY
28

SUNDAY
29

WEEKLY GOALS

MARCH 2020

MONDAY

30

TUESDAY

31

WEDNESDAY

1

THURSDAY

2

FRIDAY

3

SATURDAY

4

SUNDAY

5

WEEKLY GOALS

APRIL

Sunday	Monday	Tuesday	Wednesday
			1
5	6	7	8
12	13	14	15
19	20	21	22
26	27	28	29

Thursday	Friday	Saturday	Notes
2	**3**	**4**	
9	**10**	**11**	
16	**17**	**18**	
23	**24**	**25**	
30			

MARCH

S	M	T	W	T	F	S
1	2	3	4	5	6	7
8	9	10	11	12	13	14
15	16	17	18	19	20	21
22	23	24	25	26	27	28
29	30	31				

MAY

S	M	T	W	T	F	S
					1	2
3	4	5	6	7	8	9
10	11	12	13	14	15	16
17	18	19	20	21	22	23
24	25	26	27	28	29	30
31						

APRIL 2020

MONDAY

6

TUESDAY

7

WEDNESDAY

8

THURSDAY

9

FRIDAY

10

SATURDAY

11

SUNDAY

12

WEEKLY GOALS

APRIL 2020

MONDAY
13

TUESDAY
14

WEDNESDAY
15

THURSDAY
16

FRIDAY

17

SATURDAY

18

SUNDAY

19

WEEKLY GOALS

APRIL 2020

MONDAY

20

TUESDAY

21

WEDNESDAY

22

THURSDAY

23

FRIDAY
24

SATURDAY
25

SUNDAY
26

WEEKLY GOALS

APRIL 2020

MONDAY

27

TUESDAY

28

WEDNESDAY

29

THURSDAY

30

FRIDAY

1

SATURDAY

2

SUNDAY

3

WEEKLY GOALS

MAY

Sunday	Monday	Tuesday	Wednesday
3	4	5	6
10	11	12	13
17	18	19	20
24	25	26	27

2020

Thursday	Friday	Saturday	Notes
	1	2	
7	8	9	
14	15	16	
21	22	23	**APRIL**
28	29	30/31	**JUNE**

APRIL

S	M	T	W	T	F	S
			1	2	3	4
5	6	7	8	9	10	11
12	13	14	15	16	17	18
19	20	21	22	23	24	25
26	27	28	29	30		

JUNE

S	M	T	W	T	F	S
	1	2	3	4	5	6
7	8	9	10	11	12	13
14	15	16	17	18	19	20
21	22	23	24	25	26	27
28	29	30				

MAY 2020

MONDAY

4

TUESDAY

5

WEDNESDAY

6

THURSDAY

7

FRIDAY

8

SATURDAY

9

SUNDAY

10

WEEKLY GOALS

MAY 2020

MONDAY
11

TUESDAY
12

WEDNESDAY
13

THURSDAY
14

MAY 2020

FRIDAY
15

SATURDAY
16

SUNDAY
17

WEEKLY GOALS

MAY 2020

MONDAY
18

TUESDAY
19

WEDNESDAY
20

THURSDAY
21

FRIDAY

22

SATURDAY

23

SUNDAY

24

WEEKLY GOALS

MAY 2020

MONDAY

25

TUESDAY

26

WEDNESDAY

27

THURSDAY

28

FRIDAY
29

SATURDAY
30

SUNDAY
31

WEEKLY GOALS

JUNE

Sunday	Monday	Tuesday	Wednesday
	1	2	3
7	8	9	10
14	15	16	17
21	22	23	24
28	29	30	

Thursday	Friday	Saturday	Notes
4	5	6	
11	12	13	
18	19	20	
25	26	27	

MAY

S	M	T	W	T	F	S
					1	2
3	4	5	6	7	8	9
10	11	12	13	14	15	16
17	18	19	20	21	22	23
24	25	26	27	28	29	30
31						

JULY

S	M	T	W	T	F	S
			1	2	3	4
5	6	7	8	9	10	11
12	13	14	15	16	17	18
19	20	21	22	23	24	25
26	27	28	29	30	31	

JUNE 2020

MONDAY

1

TUESDAY

2

WEDNESDAY

3

THURSDAY

4

JUNE 2020

FRIDAY

5

SATURDAY

6

SUNDAY

7

WEEKLY GOALS

JUNE 2020

MONDAY
8

TUESDAY
9

WEDNESDAY
10

THURSDAY
11

JUNE 2020

FRIDAY

12

SATURDAY

13

SUNDAY

14

WEEKLY GOALS

JUNE 2020

MONDAY

15

TUESDAY

16

WEDNESDAY

17

THURSDAY

18

FRIDAY

19

SATURDAY

20

SUNDAY

21

WEEKLY GOALS

JUNE 2020

MONDAY
22

TUESDAY
23

WEDNESDAY
24

THURSDAY
25

FRIDAY
26

SATURDAY
27

SUNDAY
28

WEEKLY GOALS

JUNE 2020

MONDAY

29

TUESDAY

30

WEDNESDAY

1

THURSDAY

2

FRIDAY

3

SATURDAY

4

SUNDAY

5

WEEKLY GOALS

JULY

Sunday	Monday	Tuesday	Wednesday
			1
5	6	7	8
12	13	14	15
19	20	21	22
26	27	28	29

Thursday	Friday	Saturday	Notes
2	**3**	**4**	
9	**10**	**11**	
16	**17**	**18**	
23	**24**	**25**	
30	**31**		

JUNE

S	M	T	W	T	F	S
	1	2	3	4	5	6
7	8	9	10	11	12	13
14	15	16	17	18	19	20
21	22	23	24	25	26	27
28	29	30				

AUGUST

S	M	T	W	T	F	S
						1
2	3	4	5	6	7	8
9	10	11	12	13	14	15
16	17	18	19	20	21	22
23	24	25	26	27	28	29
30	31					

JULY 2020

MONDAY

6

TUESDAY

7

WEDNESDAY

8

THURSDAY

9

JULY 2020

FRIDAY
10

SATURDAY
11

SUNDAY
12

WEEKLY GOALS

JULY 2020

MONDAY

13

TUESDAY

14

WEDNESDAY

15

THURSDAY

16

FRIDAY
17

SATURDAY
18

SUNDAY
19

WEEKLY GOALS

JULY 2020

MONDAY

20

TUESDAY

21

WEDNESDAY

22

THURSDAY

23

FRIDAY

24

SATURDAY

25

SUNDAY

26

WEEKLY GOALS

JULY 2020

MONDAY

27

TUESDAY

28

WEDNESDAY

29

THURSDAY

30

AUGUST 2020

FRIDAY
31

SATURDAY
1

SUNDAY
2

WEEKLY GOALS

AUGUST

Sunday	Monday	Tuesday	Wednesday
1/2	3	4	5
9	10	11	12
16	17	18	19
23	24	25	26
30	31		

2020

Thursday	Friday	Saturday	Notes
6	**7**	**8**	
13	**14**	**15**	
20	**21**	**22**	
27	**28**	**29**	

JULY

S	M	T	W	T	F	S
			1	2	3	4
5	6	7	8	9	10	11
12	13	14	15	16	17	18
19	20	21	22	23	24	25
26	27	28	29	30	31	

SEPTEMBER

S	M	T	W	T	F	S
		1	2	3	4	5
6	7	8	9	10	11	12
13	14	15	16	17	18	19
20	21	22	23	24	25	26
27	28	29	30			

AUGUST 2020

MONDAY
3

TUESDAY
4

WEDNESDAY
5

THURSDAY
6

FRIDAY
7

SATURDAY
8

SUNDAY
9

WEEKLY GOALS

AUGUST 2020

MONDAY
10

TUESDAY
11

WEDNESDAY
12

THURSDAY
13

AUGUST 2020

FRIDAY
14

SATURDAY
15

SUNDAY
16

WEEKLY GOALS

AUGUST 2020

MONDAY
17

TUESDAY
18

WEDNESDAY
19

THURSDAY
20

AUGUST 2020

FRIDAY

21

SATURDAY

22

SUNDAY

23

WEEKLY GOALS

AUGUST 2020

MONDAY

24

TUESDAY

25

WEDNESDAY

26

THURSDAY

27

FRIDAY
28

SATURDAY
29

SUNDAY
30

WEEKLY GOALS

SEPTEMBER

Sunday	Monday	Tuesday	Wednesday
		1	2
6	7	8	9
13	14	15	16
20	21	22	23
27	28	29	30

Thursday	Friday	Saturday	Notes
3	4	5	
10	11	12	
17	18	19	
24	25	26	

AUGUST

S	M	T	W	T	F	S
						1
2	3	4	5	6	7	8
9	10	11	12	13	14	15
16	17	18	19	20	21	22
23	24	25	26	27	28	29
30	31					

OCTOBER

S	M	T	W	T	F	S
				1	2	3
4	5	6	7	8	9	10
11	12	13	14	15	16	17
18	19	20	21	22	23	24
25	26	27	28	29	30	31

SEPTEMBER 2020

MONDAY
31

TUESDAY
1

WEDNESDAY
2

THURSDAY
3

SEPTEMBER 2020

FRIDAY
4

SATURDAY
5

SUNDAY
6

WEEKLY GOALS

SEPTEMBER 2020

MONDAY

7

TUESDAY

8

WEDNESDAY

9

THURSDAY

10

SEPTEMBER 2020

FRIDAY
11

SATURDAY
12

SUNDAY
13

WEEKLY GOALS

SEPTEMBER 2020

MONDAY
14

TUESDAY
15

WEDNESDAY
16

THURSDAY
17

FRIDAY
18

SATURDAY
19

SUNDAY
20

WEEKLY GOALS

SEPTEMBER 2020

MONDAY
21

TUESDAY
22

WEDNESDAY
23

THURSDAY
24

SEPTEMBER 2020

FRIDAY
25

SATURDAY
26

SUNDAY
27

WEEKLY GOALS

SEPTEMBER 2020

MONDAY
28

TUESDAY
29

WEDNESDAY
30

THURSDAY
1

OCTOBER 2020

FRIDAY
2

SATURDAY
3

SUNDAY
4

WEEKLY GOALS

OCTOBER

Sunday	Monday	Tuesday	Wednesday
4	5	6	7
11	12	13	14
18	19	20	21
25	26	27	28

Thursday	Friday	Saturday	Notes
1	**2**	**3**	
8	**9**	**10**	
15	**16**	**17**	
22	**23**	**24**	**SEPTEMBER**
29	**30**	**31**	**NOVEMBER**

SEPTEMBER

S	M	T	W	T	F	S
		1	2	3	4	5
6	7	8	9	10	11	12
13	14	15	16	17	18	19
20	21	22	23	24	25	26
27	28	29	30			

NOVEMBER

S	M	T	W	T	F	S
1	2	3	4	5	6	7
8	9	10	11	12	13	14
15	16	17	18	19	20	21
22	23	24	25	26	27	28
29	30					

OCTOBER 2020

MONDAY

5

TUESDAY

6

WEDNESDAY

7

THURSDAY

8

OCTOBER 2020

FRIDAY
9

SATURDAY
10

SUNDAY
11

WEEKLY GOALS

SEPTEMBER 2020

MONDAY
12

TUESDAY
13

WEDNESDAY
14

THURSDAY
15

SEPTEMBER 2020

FRIDAY
16

SATURDAY
17

SUNDAY
18

WEEKLY GOALS

OCTOBER 2020

MONDAY
19

TUESDAY
20

WEDNESDAY
21

THURSDAY
22

FRIDAY

23

SATURDAY

24

SUNDAY

25

WEEKLY GOALS

OCTOBER 2020

MONDAY
26

TUESDAY
27

WEDNESDAY
28

THURSDAY
29

OCTOBER 2020

FRIDAY
30

SATURDAY
31

SUNDAY
1

WEEKLY GOALS

NOVEMBER

Sunday	Monday	Tuesday	Wednesday
1	2	3	4
8	9	10	11
15	16	17	18
22	23	24	25
29	30		

2020

Thursday	Friday	Saturday	Notes
5	**6**	**7**	
12	**13**	**14**	
19	**20**	**21**	
26	**27**	**28**	

OCTOBER

S	M	T	W	T	F	S
				1	2	3
4	5	6	7	8	9	10
11	12	13	14	15	16	17
18	19	20	21	22	23	24
25	26	27	28	29	30	31

DECEMBER

S	M	T	W	T	F	S
		1	2	3	4	5
6	7	8	9	10	11	12
13	14	15	16	17	18	19
20	21	22	23	24	25	26
27	28	29	30	31		

NOVEMBER 2020

MONDAY
2

TUESDAY
3

WEDNESDAY
4

THURSDAY
5

FRIDAY
6

SATURDAY
7

SUNDAY
8

WEEKLY GOALS

NOVEMBER 2020

MONDAY

9

TUESDAY

10

WEDNESDAY

11

THURSDAY

12

NOVEMBER 2020

FRIDAY
13

SATURDAY
14

SUNDAY
15

WEEKLY GOALS

NOVEMBER 2020

MONDAY
16

TUESDAY
17

WEDNESDAY
18

THURSDAY
19

NOVEMBER 2020

FRIDAY
20

SATURDAY
21

SUNDAY
22

WEEKLY GOALS

NOVEMBER 2020

MONDAY

23

TUESDAY

24

WEDNESDAY

25

THURSDAY

26

FRIDAY
27

SATURDAY
28

SUNDAY
29

WEEKLY GOALS

DECEMBER

Sunday	Monday	Tuesday	Wednesday
		1	2
6	7	8	9
13	14	15	16
20	21	22	23
27	28	29	30

Thursday	Friday	Saturday	Notes
3	4	5	
10	11	12	
17	18	19	
24	25	26	**NOVEMBER**
31			**JANUARY**

NOVEMBER

S	M	T	W	T	F	S
1	2	3	4	5	6	7
8	9	10	11	12	13	14
15	16	17	18	19	20	21
22	23	24	25	26	27	28
29	30					

JANUARY

S	M	T	W	T	F	S
					1	2
3	4	5	6	7	8	9
10	11	12	13	14	15	16
17	18	19	20	21	22	23
24	25	26	27	28	29	30
31						

DECEMBER 2020

MONDAY

30

TUESDAY

1

WEDNESDAY

2

THURSDAY

3

FRIDAY

4

SATURDAY

5

SUNDAY

6

WEEKLY GOALS

DECEMBER 2020

MONDAY
7

TUESDAY
18

WEDNESDAY
9

THURSDAY
10

FRIDAY
11

SATURDAY
12

SUNDAY
13

WEEKLY GOALS

DECEMBER 2020

MONDAY
14

TUESDAY
15

WEDNESDAY
16

THURSDAY
17

FRIDAY

18

SATURDAY

19

SUNDAY

20

WEEKLY GOALS

DECEMBER 2020

MONDAY
21

TUESDAY
22

WEDNESDAY
23

THURSDAY
24

DECEMBER 2020

FRIDAY
25

SATURDAY
26

SUNDAY
27

WEEKLY GOALS

DECEMBER 2020

MONDAY

28

TUESDAY

29

WEDNESDAY

30

THURSDAY

31

JANUARY 2021

FRIDAY
1

SATURDAY
2

SUNDAY
3

WEEKLY GOALS

JANUARY

Sunday	Monday	Tuesday	Wednesday
3	4	5	6
10	11	12	13
17	18	19	20
24	25	26	27

Thursday	Friday	Saturday	Notes
	1	2	
7	8	9	
14	15	16	
21	22	23	**DECEMBER**
28	29	30/31	**FEBRUARY**

DECEMBER

S	M	T	W	T	F	S
		1	2	3	4	5
6	7	8	9	10	11	12
13	14	15	16	17	18	19
20	21	22	23	24	25	26
27	28	29	30	31		

FEBRUARY

S	M	T	W	T	F	S
	1	2	3	4	5	6
7	8	9	10	11	12	13
14	15	16	17	18	19	20
21	22	23	24	25	26	27
28	29					

JANUARY 2021

MONDAY

4

TUESDAY

5

WEDNESDAY

6

THURSDAY

7

FRIDAY

8

SATURDAY

9

SUNDAY

10

WEEKLY GOALS

JANUARY 2021

MONDAY
11

TUESDAY
12

WEDNESDAY
13

THURSDAY
14

FRIDAY

15

SATURDAY

16

SUNDAY

17

WEEKLY GOALS

JANUARY 2021

MONDAY

18

TUESDAY

19

WEDNESDAY

20

THURSDAY

21

FRIDAY

22

SATURDAY

23

SUNDAY

24

WEEKLY GOALS

JANUARY 2021

MONDAY
25

TUESDAY
26

WEDNESDAY
27

THURSDAY
28

JANUARY 2021

FRIDAY

29

SATURDAY

30

SUNDAY

31

WEEKLY GOALS

FEBRUARY

Sunday	Monday	Tuesday	Wednesday
	1	2	3
7	8	9	10
14	15	16	17
21	22	23	24
28			

Thursday	Friday	Saturday	Notes
4	5	6	
11	12	13	
18	19	20	
25	26	27	

JANUARY

S	M	T	W	T	F	S
					1	2
3	4	5	6	7	8	9
10	11	12	13	14	15	16
17	18	19	20	21	22	23
24	25	26	27	28	29	30
31						

MARCH

S	M	T	W	T	F	S
	1	2	3	4	5	6
7	8	9	10	11	12	13
14	15	16	17	18	19	20
21	22	23	24	25	26	27
28	29	30	31			

FEBRUARY 2021

MONDAY
1

TUESDAY
2

WEDNESDAY
3

THURSDAY
4

FEBRUARY 2021

FRIDAY
5

SATURDAY
6

SUNDAY
7

WEEKLY GOALS

FEBRUARY 2021

MONDAY
8

TUESDAY
9

WEDNESDAY
10

THURSDAY
11

FEBRUARY 2021

FRIDAY

12

SATURDAY

13

SUNDAY

14

WEEKLY GOALS

FEBRUARY 2021

MONDAY
15

TUESDAY
16

WEDNESDAY
17

THURSDAY
18

FRIDAY

19

SATURDAY

20

SUNDAY

21

WEEKLY GOALS

FEBRUARY 2021

MONDAY
22

TUESDAY
23

WEDNESDAY
24

THURSDAY
25

FRIDAY
26

SATURDAY
27

SUNDAY
28

WEEKLY GOALS

MARCH

Sunday	Monday	Tuesday	Wednesday
	1	2	3
7	8	9	10
14	15	16	17
21	22	23	24
28	29	30	31

Thursday	Friday	Saturday	Notes
4	5	6	
11	12	13	
18	19	20	
25	26	27	

FEBRUARY

S	M	T	W	T	F	S
	1	2	3	4	5	6
7	8	9	10	11	12	13
14	15	16	17	18	19	20
21	22	23	24	25	26	27
28	29					

APRIL

S	M	T	W	T	F	S
				1	2	3
4	5	6	7	8	9	10
11	12	13	14	15	16	17
18	19	20	21	22	23	24
25	26	27	28	29	30	

MARCH 2021

MONDAY

1

TUESDAY

2

WEDNESDAY

3

THURSDAY

4

FRIDAY

5

SATURDAY

6

SUNDAY

7

WEEKLY GOALS

MARCH 2021

MONDAY
8

TUESDAY
9

WEDNESDAY
10

THURSDAY
11

FRIDAY
12

SATURDAY
13

SUNDAY
14

WEEKLY GOALS

MARCH 2021

MONDAY

15

TUESDAY

16

WEDNESDAY

17

THURSDAY

18

FRIDAY
19

SATURDAY
20

SUNDAY
21

WEEKLY GOALS

MARCH 2021

MONDAY

22

TUESDAY

23

WEDNESDAY

24

THURSDAY

25

FRIDAY
26

SATURDAY
27

SUNDAY
28

WEEKLY GOALS

MARCH 2021

MONDAY
29

TUESDAY
30

WEDNESDAY
31

THURSDAY
1

FRIDAY

2

SATURDAY

3

SUNDAY

4

WEEKLY GOALS

APRIL

Sunday	Monday	Tuesday	Wednesday
4	5	6	7
11	12	13	14
18	19	20	21
25	26	27	28

Thursday	Friday	Saturday	Notes
1	2	3	
8	9	10	
15	16	17	
22	23	24	**MARCH**
29	30		**MAY**

MARCH

S	M	T	W	T	F	S
	1	2	3	4	5	6
7	8	9	10	11	12	13
14	15	16	17	18	19	20
21	22	23	24	25	26	27
28	29	30	31			

MAY

S	M	T	W	T	F	S
						1
2	3	4	5	6	7	8
9	10	11	12	13	14	15
16	17	18	19	20	21	22
23	24	25	26	27	28	29
30	31					

APRIL 2021

MONDAY
5

TUESDAY
6

WEDNESDAY
7

THURSDAY
8

FRIDAY

9

SATURDAY

10

SUNDAY

11

WEEKLY GOALS

APRIL 2021

MONDAY
12

TUESDAY
13

WEDNESDAY
14

THURSDAY
15

FRIDAY

16

SATURDAY

17

SUNDAY

18

WEEKLY GOALS

APRIL 2021

MONDAY

19

TUESDAY

20

WEDNESDAY

21

THURSDAY

22

FRIDAY
23

SATURDAY
24

SUNDAY
25

WEEKLY GOALS

APRIL 2021

MONDAY
26

TUESDAY
27

WEDNESDAY
28

THURSDAY
29

FRIDAY
30

SATURDAY
1

SUNDAY
2

WEEKLY GOALS

MAY

Sunday	Monday	Tuesday	Wednesday
1/2	3	4	5
9	10	11	12
16	17	18	19
23	24	25	26
30	31		

Thursday	Friday	Saturday	Notes
6	**7**	**8**	
13	**14**	**15**	
20	**21**	**22**	
27	**28**	**29**	**APRIL**

APRIL

S	M	T	W	T	F	S
				1	2	3
4	5	6	7	8	9	10
11	12	13	14	15	16	17
18	19	20	21	22	23	24
25	26	27	28	29	30	

JUNE

S	M	T	W	T	F	S
		1	2	3	4	5
6	7	8	9	10	11	12
13	14	15	16	17	18	19
20	21	22	23	24	25	26
27	28	29	30			

MAY 2021

MONDAY
3

TUESDAY
4

WEDNESDAY
5

THURSDAY
6

MAY 2021

FRIDAY
7

SATURDAY
8

SUNDAY
9

WEEKLY GOALS

MAY 2021

MONDAY
10

TUESDAY
11

WEDNESDAY
12

THURSDAY
13

FRIDAY
14

SATURDAY
15

SUNDAY
16

WEEKLY GOALS

MAY 2021

MONDAY

17

TUESDAY

18

WEDNESDAY

19

THURSDAY

20

FRIDAY
21

SATURDAY
22

SUNDAY
23

WEEKLY GOALS

MAY 2021

MONDAY

24

TUESDAY

25

WEDNESDAY

26

THURSDAY

27

FRIDAY

28

SATURDAY

29

SUNDAY

30

WEEKLY GOALS

JUNE

Sunday	Monday	Tuesday	Wednesday
		1	2
6	7	8	9
13	14	15	16
20	21	22	23
27	28	29	30

Thursday	Friday	Saturday	Notes
3	**4**	**5**	
10	**11**	**12**	
17	**18**	**19**	
24	**25**	**26**	**MAY**

MAY

S	M	T	W	T	F	S
						1
2	3	4	5	6	7	8
9	10	11	12	13	14	15
16	17	18	19	20	21	22
23	24	25	26	27	28	29
30	31					

JULY

S	M	T	W	T	F	S
				1	2	3
4	5	6	7	8	9	10
11	12	13	14	15	16	17
18	19	20	21	22	23	24
25	26	27	28	29	30	31

JUNE 2021

MONDAY
31

TUESDAY
1

WEDNESDAY
2

THURSDAY
3

FRIDAY

4

SATURDAY

5

SUNDAY

6

WEEKLY GOALS

JUNE 2021

MONDAY
7

TUESDAY
8

WEDNESDAY
9

THURSDAY
10

FRIDAY
11

SATURDAY
12

SUNDAY
13

WEEKLY GOALS

JUNE 2021

MONDAY

14

TUESDAY

15

WEDNESDAY

16

THURSDAY

17

FRIDAY
18

SATURDAY
19

SUNDAY
20

WEEKLY GOALS

JUNE 2021

MONDAY
21

TUESDAY
22

WEDNESDAY
23

THURSDAY
24

JUNE 2021

FRIDAY
25

SATURDAY
26

SUNDAY
27

WEEKLY GOALS

JUNE 2021

MONDAY
28

TUESDAY
29

WEDNESDAY
30

THURSDAY
1

FRIDAY

2

SATURDAY

3

SUNDAY

4

WEEKLY GOALS

JULY

Sunday	Monday	Tuesday	Wednesday
4	5	6	7
11	12	13	14
18	19	20	21
25	26	27	28

Thursday	Friday	Saturday	Notes
1	2	3	
8	9	10	
15	16	17	
22	23	24	
29	30	31	

JUNE

S	M	T	W	T	F	S
		1	2	3	4	5
6	7	8	9	10	11	12
13	14	15	16	17	18	19
20	21	22	23	24	25	26
27	28	29	30			

AUGUST

S	M	T	W	T	F	S
1	2	3	4	5	6	7
8	9	10	11	12	13	14
15	16	17	18	19	20	21
22	23	24	25	26	27	28
29	30	31				

JULY 2021

MONDAY
5

TUESDAY
6

WEDNESDAY
7

THURSDAY
8

FRIDAY

9

SATURDAY

10

SUNDAY

11

WEEKLY GOALS

JULY 2021

MONDAY
12

TUESDAY
13

WEDNESDAY
14

THURSDAY
15

FRIDAY

16

SATURDAY

17

SUNDAY

18

WEEKLY GOALS

JULY 2021

MONDAY
19

TUESDAY
20

WEDNESDAY
21

THURSDAY
22

FRIDAY

23

SATURDAY

24

SUNDAY

25

WEEKLY GOALS

JULY 2021

MONDAY

26

TUESDAY

27

WEDNESDAY

28

THURSDAY

29

FRIDAY
30

SATURDAY
31

SUNDAY
1

WEEKLY GOALS

AUGUST

Sunday	Monday	Tuesday	Wednesday
1	2	3	4
8	9	10	11
15	16	17	18
22	23	24	25
29	30	31	

2021

Thursday	Friday	Saturday	Notes
5	**6**	**7**	
12	**13**	**14**	
19	**20**	**21**	
26	**27**	**28**	JULY

JULY

S	M	T	W	T	F	S
				1	2	3
4	5	6	7	8	9	10
11	12	13	14	15	16	17
18	19	20	21	22	23	24
25	26	27	28	29	30	31

SEPTEMBER

S	M	T	W	T	F	S
			1	2	3	4
5	6	7	8	9	10	11
12	13	14	15	16	17	18
19	20	21	22	23	24	25
26	27	28	29	30		

AUGUST 2021

MONDAY
2

TUESDAY
3

WEDNESDAY
4

THURSDAY
5

FRIDAY

6

SATURDAY

7

SUNDAY

8

WEEKLY GOALS

AUGUST 2021

MONDAY
9

TUESDAY
10

WEDNESDAY
11

THURSDAY
12

FRIDAY
13

SATURDAY
14

SUNDAY
15

WEEKLY GOALS

AUGUST 2021

MONDAY
16

TUESDAY
17

WEDNESDAY
18

THURSDAY
19

FRIDAY
20

SATURDAY
21

SUNDAY
22

WEEKLY GOALS

AUGUST 2021

MONDAY
23

TUESDAY
24

WEDNESDAY
25

THURSDAY
26

FRIDAY

27

SATURDAY

28

SUNDAY

29

WEEKLY GOALS

AUGUST 2021

MONDAY

30

TUESDAY

31

WEDNESDAY

1

THURSDAY

2

FRIDAY

3

SATURDAY

4

SUNDAY

5

WEEKLY GOALS

SEPTEMBER

Sunday	Monday	Tuesday	Wednesday
			1
5	6	7	8
12	13	14	15
19	20	21	22
26	27	28	29

Thursday	Friday	Saturday	Notes
2	3	4	
9	10	11	
16	17	18	
23	24	25	
30			

AUGUST

S	M	T	W	T	F	S
1	2	3	4	5	6	7
8	9	10	11	12	13	14
15	16	17	18	19	20	21
22	23	24	25	26	27	28
29	30	31				

OCTOBER

S	M	T	W	T	F	S
					1	2
3	4	5	6	7	8	9
10	11	12	13	14	15	16
17	18	19	20	21	22	23
24	25	26	27	28	29	30
31						

SEPTEMBER 2021

MONDAY

6

TUESDAY

7

WEDNESDAY

8

THURSDAY

9

FRIDAY
10

SATURDAY
11

SUNDAY
12

WEEKLY GOALS

SEPTEMBER 2021

MONDAY
13

TUESDAY
14

WEDNESDAY
15

THURSDAY
16

SEPTEMBER 2021

FRIDAY
17

SATURDAY
18

SUNDAY
19

WEEKLY GOALS

SEPTEMBER 2021

MONDAY
20

TUESDAY
21

WEDNESDAY
22

THURSDAY
23

FRIDAY

24

SATURDAY

25

SUNDAY

26

WEEKLY GOALS

SEPTEMBER 2021

MONDAY
27

TUESDAY
28

WEDNESDAY
29

THURSDAY
30

FRIDAY

1

SATURDAY

2

SUNDAY

3

WEEKLY GOALS

OCTOBER

Sunday	Monday	Tuesday	Wednesday
3	4	5	6
10	11	12	13
17	18	19	20
24	25	26	27

2021

Thursday	Friday	Saturday	Notes
	1	2	
7	8	9	
14	15	16	
21	22	23	
28	29	30/31	

SEPTEMBER

S	M	T	W	T	F	S
			1	2	3	4
5	6	7	8	9	10	11
12	13	14	15	16	17	18
19	20	21	22	23	24	25
26	27	28	29	30		

NOVEMBER

S	M	T	W	T	F	S
	1	2	3	4	5	6
7	8	9	10	11	12	13
14	15	16	17	18	19	20
21	22	23	24	25	26	27
28	29	30				

OCTOBER 2021

MONDAY
4

TUESDAY
5

WEDNESDAY
6

THURSDAY
7

FRIDAY

8

SATURDAY

9

SUNDAY

10

WEEKLY GOALS

OCTOBER 2021

MONDAY
11

TUESDAY
12

WEDNESDAY
13

THURSDAY
14

OCTOBER 2021

FRIDAY

15

SATURDAY

16

SUNDAY

17

WEEKLY GOALS

OCTOBER 2021

MONDAY
18

TUESDAY
19

WEDNESDAY
20

THURSDAY
21

OCTOBER 2021

FRIDAY
22

SATURDAY
23

SUNDAY
24

WEEKLY GOALS

OCTOBER 2021

MONDAY
25

TUESDAY
26

WEDNESDAY
27

THURSDAY
28

FRIDAY

29

SATURDAY

30

SUNDAY

31

WEEKLY GOALS

NOVEMBER

Sunday	Monday	Tuesday	Wednesday
	1	2	3
7	8	9	10
14	15	16	17
21	22	23	24
28	29	30	

Thursday	Friday	Saturday	Notes
4	5	6	
11	12	13	
18	19	20	
25	26	27	

OCTOBER

S	M	T	W	T	F	S
					1	2
3	4	5	6	7	8	9
10	11	12	13	14	15	16
17	18	19	20	21	22	23
24	25	26	27	28	29	30
31						

DECEMBER

S	M	T	W	T	F	S
			1	2	3	4
5	6	7	8	9	10	11
12	13	14	15	16	17	18
19	20	21	22	23	24	25
26	27	28	29	30	31	

NOVEMBER 2021

MONDAY
1

TUESDAY
2

WEDNESDAY
3

THURSDAY
4

FRIDAY

5

SATURDAY

6

SUNDAY

7

WEEKLY GOALS

NOVEMBER 2021

MONDAY
8

TUESDAY
9

WEDNESDAY
10

THURSDAY
11

FRIDAY

12

SATURDAY

13

SUNDAY

14

WEEKLY GOALS

NOVEMBER 2021

MONDAY

15

TUESDAY

16

WEDNESDAY

17

THURSDAY

18

NOVEMBER 2021

FRIDAY

19

SATURDAY

20

SUNDAY

21

WEEKLY GOALS

NOVEMBER 2021

MONDAY
22

TUESDAY
23

WEDNESDAY
24

THURSDAY
25

FRIDAY

26

SATURDAY

27

SUNDAY

28

WEEKLY GOALS

NOVEMBER 2021

MONDAY

29

TUESDAY

30

WEDNESDAY

1

THURSDAY

2

DECEMBER 2021

FRIDAY
3

SATURDAY
4

SUNDAY
5

WEEKLY GOALS

DECEMBER

Sunday	Monday	Tuesday	Wednesday
			1
5	6	7	8
12	13	14	15
19	20	21	22
26	27	28	29

Thursday	Friday	Saturday	Notes
2	3	4	
9	10	11	
16	17	18	
23	24	25	
30	31		

NOVEMBER

S	M	T	W	T	F	S
	1	2	3	4	5	6
7	8	9	10	11	12	13
14	15	16	17	18	19	20
21	22	23	24	25	26	27
28	29	30				

JANUARY

S	M	T	W	T	F	S
						1
2	3	4	5	6	7	8
9	10	11	12	13	14	15
16	17	18	19	20	21	22
23	24	25	26	27	28	29
30	31					

DECEMBER 2021

MONDAY

6

TUESDAY

7

WEDNESDAY

8

THURSDAY

9

DECEMBER 2021

FRIDAY
10

SATURDAY
11

SUNDAY
12

WEEKLY GOALS

DECEMBER 2021

MONDAY
13

TUESDAY
14

WEDNESDAY
15

THURSDAY
16

DECEMBER 2021

FRIDAY

17

SATURDAY

18

SUNDAY

19

WEEKLY GOALS

DECEMBER 2021

MONDAY
20

TUESDAY
21

WEDNESDAY
22

THURSDAY
23

FRIDAY

24

SATURDAY

25

SUNDAY

26

WEEKLY GOALS

DECEMBER 2021

MONDAY
27

TUESDAY
28

WEDNESDAY
29

THURSDAY
30

DECEMBER 2021

FRIDAY
31

SATURDAY
1

SUNDAY
2

WEEKLY GOALS

Made in the USA
Las Vegas, NV
24 April 2025

21319969R00149